Curing
MERALGIA
PARESTHETICA

Godfree Roberts, Ed.D.

Published by

Table of Contents

Contents

LAURA'S STORY

I'm 30 yrs old. I began suffering from Meralgia when I was 3 month pregnant. My baby is now 7 months and I still have it. I lost all my weight which was really insignificant.

I don't have the pins and needles, but the numbness is there and when I overdo it I get the burning sensation still. When I say "overdo it" I mean go shopping, cook, or drive for more than half hour!!!

I tried cortisone injection, chiropractic, the cat-cow exercises, swimming, resting, massaging, ice, sleeping with special pillow, taking medication, taking vitamins...YOU NAME IT!!

My neurologist discouraged swimming, as this nerve is so superficial that can be pressured from the water itself!

*I have to admit that it's not as bad, but **I have come to the conclusion that nerve conditions take a lot of time and conservative measures are the key**.*

My neurologist says that the nerves recover on their own by 1 millimeter per day so...do the math! Unfortunately it's a condition that can be caused by many parameters...

This message goes to the future Docs out there: If I were a doctor I would definitely do my PhD on this! You would definitely win a Nobel Prize or something!!

Thanks for listening!
Ciao, Laura

WHAT IS MERALGIA PARESTHETICA?

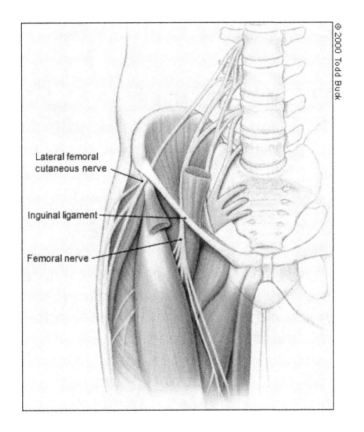

Lateral femoral cutaneous nerve

Inguinal ligament

Femoral nerve

© 2000 Todd Buck

This illustration of the LFCN is by one of the world's
leading anatomical illustrators, Todd Buck.
Anyone
interested in the human body will enjoy his
work.

Meralgia paresthetica (MP) is a condition characterized by numbness, tingling, pain or burning along the outer thigh which can extend from the hip and buttock to the knee. It occurs when the lateral femoral cutaneous nerve (LFCN) – which supplies sensation to the outer thigh – is compressed or trapped at the point where it exits the pelvis.

ANATOMY

The lateral femoral cutaneous nerve exits the spine as a variable and complex bundle of nerve fibers. It arises from various and changeable locations in the spinal column and takes a variety of ways to get to your thigh. Here's how it is usually described in anatomy texts:

> *The LFCN is primarily a sensory nerve but also includes efferent sympathetic fibers carrying vasomotor, pilomotor, and sudomotor impulses. It is quite variable and may be derived from several different combinations of lumbar nerves, including L2 and L3, L1 and L2, L2 alone, and L3 alone. The LFCN may be associated with the femoral nerve as it passes through the inguinal ligament or may anastomose with the femoral nerve distal to the inguinal ligament. Piersol reported that the LFCN may be partially or entirely derived from the adjacent genitofemoral or femoral nerve, and*

Keegan and Holyoke noted this variation in 30% of their cadaver dissections. On occasion, the LFCN is absent and may be replaced by a branch of the ilioinguinal nerve.

The LFCN passes behind the psoas muscle and runs beneath the iliac fascia as it crosses the surface of the iliacus muscle. As the nerve approaches the anterior superior iliac spine, it pierces the iliac fascia and exits through a fibrous tunnel into the thigh. Roth noted that the nerve is vulnerable to pressure or stretching where it emerges beneath the psoas muscle, passes around the anterior superior iliac spine, courses through the fibrous canal of the fascia lata, and finally exits the fascia lata. The site at which the LFCN exits the pelvis varies, and symptoms of meralgia paresthetica have been reported with each of five known variants.

The LFCN is most frequently found passing through the split lateral attachment of the inguinal ligament. As the nerve curves medially and inferiorly around the anterior superior iliac spine, it may be subjected to repetitive trauma in this fibroosseous tunnel. Nathan observed thickening of the LFCN at this level in 60% of his cadaver dissections and postulated that this was a direct response to chronic irritation.

The nerve may pass posterior to the inguinal ligament and anterior to a sharp ridge of iliacus fascia. Ghent noted that this variation may lead to a bowstring deformity of the nerve when the patient is supine.

Occasionally, the LFCN enters the thigh within or beneath the substance of the sartorius muscle. Stookey reported that in some instances the nerve passed through a shallow bony groove posterior to the sartorius. Ghent and Stookey both reported symptomatic patients with this variation.

Several cases have been reported in which the LFCN crosses over the iliac crest lateral and posterior to the anterior superior iliac spine. The nerve typically lies in a groove in the ilium and is subject to pressure from tight garments or belts. Hager's initial case report involved this location.

The nerve may exit the pelvis in multiple branches with entrapment of a single branch. Williams and Trzil reported displacement of the branches as much as 6 cm medial to the anterior superior iliac *spine.http://www.ncbi.nlm.nih.gov/pmc /articles/PMC1421141/*

The nerve root exits your spinal cord between the lowest (twelfth) thoracic vertebra (T12) and your highest (first) lumbar vertebra (L1). It comes close to the skin when it exits from under the inguinal ligament. – Annals of Surgery.

Medical Terminology

The term *Meralgia Paraesthetica* comprises four Greek roots, which together express "thigh pain with anomalous perception". In other words, *you perceive the pain not at the point of injury to the nerve, but somewhere else* – where the nerve ends. The condition is also called *Bernhardt-Roth Syndrome, Neuralgia Paraesthetica, Femoral Cutaneous Nerve syndrome, LFCN Syndrome, Burning Thigh Syndrome.*

Demographics, Occurrence and Frequency

1. Approximately 4 cases of Meralgia paresthetica are reported in every 10,000 general clinic patients, or **3 million new cases annually** worldwide. You are not alone.

2. It occurs in 20% - 35% of patients referred for leg discomfort.

3. Up to 20% of MP patients have bilateral symptoms: the pain occurs in both legs.

4. Meralgia paresthetica is observed in all age groups but most commonly in middle-aged men.

5. The point of pressure or entrapment is usually *where the nerve exits the pelvis*, running through the inguinal ligament. But – we'll get to this later in the book – it is also worth paying attention to the vertebral joint in our spines *where the nerve exits the spinal column*.

Diagnosis

The diagnosis is usually evident based on your experience of symptoms and a simple physical examination. Neurological testing usually reveals normal thigh-muscle strength and normal reflexes, but there will be numbness or extreme sensitivity of the skin along the outer thigh.

Treatment

Apart from prescribing anti-inflammatories and painkillers, conventional medical care offers little help to MP sufferers. Depending on its severity, Meralgia paresthetica may be treated by a family MD, internal medicine specialist, neurologist, or orthopedic surgeon. But most treatment, and even diagnosis, is done by sufferers themselves.

Patients with MP are advised to lose weight and wear loose, light clothing.

In patients with *severe* pain, temporary relief can be obtained by injecting lidocaine (a local anesthetic) and steroids (an anti-inflammatory agent) into the lateral femoral cutaneous nerve.

In cases that don't respond to other treatments, surgery to free the entrapped lateral femoral cutaneous nerve may be advised in order to improve symptoms. However, surgery is a last resort. Read the chapter, below, on surgery before you commit to this approach and try everything else first.

Prognosis

The most acute pain usually lasts about 6 weeks. This can be reduced by using the treatments described in this book.

Most cases resolve themselves spontaneously within two years of the first appearance of symptoms. This book is about what you can do to gain relief from your symptoms during that time and speed your full recovery.

The treatments given here will help relieve your pain and speed your recovery. We prefer natural approaches but pharmaceuticals are often essential at onset of your symptoms.

If you have a question, have novel symptoms of MP, or find a treatment or exercise that provides relief, please let me know by emailing godfree@gmail.com.
I'll update this book so that everyone can benefit from your discovery.

WHAT CAUSES MERALGIA?

When the LFCN nerve is squeezed, crushed, swollen, or damaged it causes pain or numbness in your thigh. Caregivers may not know exactly what caused your MP. Causes can include:

- Diabetes
- Fluid buildup in the abdomen
- Lupus
- Sarcoidosis
- Acquired immunodeficiency syndrome (AIDS).
- Hip or knee arthritis
- Back pain
- Lead poisoning
- Drinking too much alcohol, too often.
- Growths in organs that are near your LFCN
- Pregnancy or growths in your uterus
- Obesity
- One leg that is longer than the other (this can usually be corrected)
- Wearing tight clothing, belts, tight-fitting leg braces that put pressure on your LFCN

- Trauma: surface or deep injuries to your thigh or groin area may cause MP.
- Leprosy (skin disease)
- Bone growth in soft tissue after an injury.
- Anti-rejection medicine that is given after an organ transplant.

If you have a question, have novel symptoms of MP, or find a treatment or exercise that provides relief, please let me know by emailing godfree@gmail.com. I'll update this book so that everyone can benefit from your discovery.

SYMPTOMS OF MERALGIA

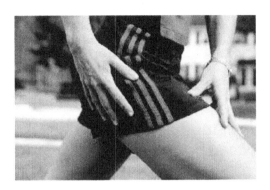

You May Experience Some or All of These:

- Pain, numbness, tingling, burning, stinging, cooling, itching or aching in the front and outer thigh, groin, buttocks *not* caused by injury to the thigh.

- Lower back/hip pain that goes down your legs.

- Multiple bee-sting like pains.

- Pain when your thigh is touched or tapped *lightly*.

- Hyper-sensitivity to heat: warm water from showering may feel like burning.

- Heightened sensitivity to touch in the outer thigh.

- Usually – 80% of the time – occurring on only one side of the body.

- Numbness in the outer thigh *or* calf.

- The skin of the outer thigh may be painfully sensitive to touch
- Pain anywhere from your hip, groin, buttocks, knee, that tends to move around.
- Pain comes and goes, usually strongest at night and diminishes by day.
- Constant weakness in your affected leg.
- Hair loss on your thigh, perhaps because you are rubbing it to decrease the pain.
- Pain or numbness may worsen if you sit and straighten your leg, or stand for long.
- Sitting may relieve your pain.
- Lying on your back with your leg raised may relieve your pain.

Note: Meralgia paresthetica should normally *not* be associated with pain radiating from the back.

*If you have a question, have novel symptoms of MP, or find a treatment or exercise
that provides relief, please let me know by emailing godfree@gmail.com.
I'll update this book so that everyone can benefit from your discovery.*

EMERGENCY TREATMENT

of Meralgia Paresthetica

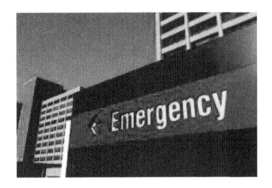

If you have a fresh case of Meralgia Paresthetica and your outer thigh, hip, back/knee are hurting badly, make an appointment to see your doctor. Then:

1. Take 300 mgm. of Gabapentin (or equivalent) every 4 hours.

2. Take 50 mgm Neofenac (diclofenac sodium or equivalent), then 25 mg. every 6 hours.

3. Wrap some ice in a thick hand towel and apply it to your inguinal region, moving it back and forth slowly. Do the same for the L1-T12 area of your spine.

4. Do the same with a HOT washcloth. Alternate the hot/cold treatments.

5. Apply a small dab of Capsaicin cream (an over-the-counter product from your pharmacist) to your inguinal region, rubbing it in until it disappears. Keep a moist washcloth handy in case it stings your skin too much. ***Do not get it on your genitals***. Wash your hands immediately after applying it. Re-apply the cream every 3-4 hours. It has no side-effects and you will not develop a tolerance: it keeps on working.

6. As you're lying down, rotate your tailbone in tiny circles, using your abdominal muscles to control the movement. Do this whenever you remember to.

7. Do the Yoga Bridge (see the Exercise page) slowly and gently, only lifting your spine up about halfway off the bed or floor, then laying it back down *one vertebra at a time*. Use your abdominal muscles to control this.

8. Make an appointment with a Chinese acupuncturist. Acupuncture is an effective treatment for most MP symptoms.

9. Rest. Lie on your back with your feet on the floor or bed. If you want to sleep on your side, place a pillow between your legs. This lessens the 'pull' on your hip muscles.

10. Can't sleep? Listen to a boring podcast of Etruscan history, or to the Buddha Machine (an

Apple iTunes app). Podcasts are one of the best ways of distracting yourself from the pain. Cheap, in-ear 'ear buds' are best for this purpose as they allow you to fall asleep without discomfort. When you buy them make sure that they do not project out far from your ear. That will allow you to fall asleep while lying on your side.

11. There's much more you can do to suppress the pain and help you recover in three weeks instead of six. Read the rest of this book and follow the simple instructions.

If you have a question, have novel symptoms of MP, or find a treatment or exercise that provides relief, please let me know by emailing godfree@gmail.com.
I'll update this book so that everyone can benefit from your discovery.

NIGHT TIME STRATEGIES FOR MERALGIA

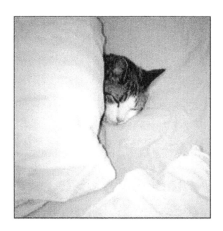

Here's an evening regime to help you sleep and not wake up feeling dopey:

First Night
1. Take one 300 mg. Gabapentin (or equivalent, according to your doctor's recommendation) *8 hours before bedtime.*

2. Take another 300 mg. Gabapentin *4 hours before bedtime.*

3. Take another 300 mg Gabapentin *just before you lie down*, along with 3 Neofenac (diclofenac sodium) 25 mg. (more, if your doctor

recommends it).

4. Get down on the floor and do the Finger-Walking Child's Pose exercise (see Exercises)

5. Just before you tuck yourself in, apply Capsaicin cream, as directed above, to you inguinal region.

Second Night
1. If the first night worked well, consider taking just two Gabapentin on the second night: one 4 hours before bedtime, and the other plus two Neofenac painkillers as you go to sleep.

2. Get down on the floor and do the Finger-Walking Child's Pose exercise (see Exercises chapter)

3. Just before you tuck yourself in, apply your Capsaicin cream, as directed, to you inguinal region.

4. This second-night drug regime can be safely maintained thereafter.

In Bed
1. Do the low, gentle version of the yoga "Bridge" as shown on the Exercises page) while lying on your back in bed.

2. Do a 360-degree rotation of your tailbone while keeping your spine still. Start out slowly tracing tiny circles with the tip of your tailbone – barely visible to an observer – and work your way up to larger circles, always moving slowly and deliberately.

3. Sleep on your side with a pillow between your legs. This keeps your knees apart and reduces tension on your hip.

4. *If you stay in bed the pain seems to get worse.* So swing your legs over the side of the bed and sit up. Get up, apply your capsaicin cream, and do the Yoga Child's Pose + Finger Walk (see the Exercises page). This helps dispel any residual night pain and allows you to start your day without more drugs.

Midnight Tricks

1. If you wake up in pain during the night, *do not* just lie there focusing on your pain.

2. Sit upright on the edge of your bed (this really helps).

3. Take another painkiller if it's 3-4 hours since the last one.

4. Wrap some ice in a washcloth or hand towel and apply it to your inguinal region, your L2-L3 lumbar region, and the area where you are currently feeling pain. That will diminish the

pain *and* distract you from focusing on it, which is almost as good.

5. Do alternating cold and hot cloth compresses. This can be most effective.

6. Drink something soothing like hot milk or Valerian tea with honey.

7. Use the Buddha Machine (Apple iTunes app) or any soothing noise generator.

Morning Routine

1. When you wake up in the morning, move around slowly and carefully.

2. Make yourself a large cup of strong Irish Breakfast tea with milk and sugar (coffee's fine, too, but harder on your digestion). This lifts your spirits and diminishes your perception of pain.

3. While your tea or coffee is brewing, get down on the floor and do the Finger-Walking Child's Pose exercise SLOWLY, GENTLY, AND COMPLETELY.

If you have a question, have novel symptoms of MP, or find a treatment or exercise that provides relief, please let me know by emailing godfree@gmail.com.

I'll update this book so that everyone can benefit from your discovery.

DRUGS FOR MERALGIA

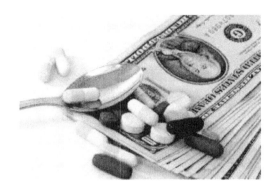

Painkillers

Medications for treatment of Meralgia paresthetica (MP) discomfort include nonsteroidal anti-inflammatory drugs (NSAIDs), narcotics, and other agents such as amitriptyline, Neurontin, and Tegretol.

Some physicians aggressively prescribe painkillers and some will not. In general, avoid prolonged use of NSAIDs and narcotics. Here are some suggestions for initiating chemical treatment for MP. Again, your experience with these and other drugs is very important to all MP sufferers, so please let us know if you discover anything we haven't covered here.

The painkillers I recommend here not only greatly reduce pain from MP, they also create drowsiness at night and allow 8 hours sleep, making additional sleeping pills unnecessary. In addition, GABA drugs produce euphoria in the morning, which provides a welcome break.

Gabapentin
My favorite is Sandoz 300 mg. Gabapentin. Its action is fairly subtle but is has four advantages:

1. It doesn't leave you feeling hungover.

2. It makes you feel euphoric until noon the next day. There's no reaction in the afternoon; the euphoria simply fades. "GABA Euphoria" is a well-known phenomenon in medicine.

3. It's non-habit forming.

4. It helps you sleep and avoid sleeping pills.

Neofenac
Neofenac is a brand name for Diclofenac, a non-steroidal anti-inflammatory drug (NSAID). It works by reducing substances in the body that cause pain inflammation. I used it because my local pharmacist recommended it (I live in Thailand where pharmacists do most diagnosing and prescribing) and it worked. If you have a recommendation for another painkiller that and knocks out the pain for 6-8 hours, let us know.

Diclofenac Potassium (Neofenac) is usually prescribed 50 mg orally 3 times a day.

In some patients an initial dose of 100 mg of diclofenac followed by 50 mg doses provides better relief. After the first day, the total daily dose generally should not (and need not, if you use the regime suggested in this website) exceed 150 mg.

Diclofenac Potassium liquid filled capsules, Zipsor®, are only approved by the FDA for mild to moderate acute pain. The dosage for this product is 25 mg orally 4 times a day.

Lidoderm Patch
Some people get relief from repeated application of Lidoderm patches. Talk to your doctor or, better still, your neurologist.

Sleeping Pills
Sleeping pills should not be necessary if you use the combination recommended above, along with the evening and morning regimes. But just in case, here's some information about them:

Some newer medications don't have the same chemical structure as a benzodiazepine (called Non-benzodiazepine sedative hypnotic sleeping pills), but act on the same area in the brain. They are thought to have fewer side effects and less risk of dependency but are still controlled substances. They include

- zalepon (Sonata)
- zolpidem (Ambien)
- eszopiclone (Lunesta) which has been tested for longer-term use, up to six months.

Based on friends' experiences with benzodiazepines I strongly recommend using them as a last resort as they can be highly addictive.

Drawbacks of Non-Benzodiazepine Sleeping Pills

Generally, non-benzodiazepines have fewer drawbacks than benzodiazepines, but that doesn't make them suitable for everyone. Some may find this type of sleep medication ineffective at helping them sleep, while the long-term effects remain unknown. Side-effects include:

- Morning grogginess
- Drug tolerance
- Rebound insomnia
- Headaches, dizziness, nausea
- Dangerous sleep-related behaviors like sleep-walking, -driving, and -eating
- More information on sleeping pills here...

If you have a question, have novel symptoms of MP, or find a treatment or exercise

that provides relief, please let me know by emailing godfree@gmail.com.
I'll update this book so that everyone can benefit from your discovery.

NATURAL TREATMENTS

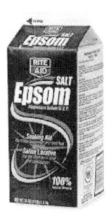

Icing
Experiment with icing L2-L3 and your inguinal region: Wrap some crushed ice in a thick hand towel and apply it gently and repeatedly to your spine and groin.

Heating
A hot, moist towel applied to the L2-L3 region and the inguinal region: apply it gently and repeatedly to your spine. You can also apply it to your inguinal region and to the painful area of your hip, thigh, or leg.

Epsom Salts Bath
Take an Epsom Salt bath with a follow-through of icing the L2-L3. Epsom salts is a common mineral salt called magnesium sulfate. When magnesium sulfate is absorbed through the skin,

such as in a bath, it draws toxins from the body, sedates the nervous system, reduces swelling, relaxes muscles, and is a natural emollient, exfoliator, and much more. *For a relaxing and sedative bath,* Soak in warm water and 2 cups of Epsom salt.

Capsaicin
Capsaicin is the active component of chili peppers, plants belonging to the genus Capsicum. It is an irritant for mammals, including humans, and can produce a sensation of burning when applied to the skin. But, when applied topically (to your skin) it, for reasons still unknown, RELIEVES PAIN. Before using capsaicin, tell your doctor about

- broken skin
- skin irritation
- previous allergic reactions to capsaicin, hot peppers
- breastfeeding
- pregnancy or current attempts to become pregnant

Buy a tube of capsaicin cream over the counter and follow the directions by rubbing a small amount into your skin where the nerve exits below the inguinal ligament, and at the L2-L3 joint area. Keep a soapy wash cloth handy in case you're supersensitive. In 5 minutes you'll start feeling relief which will last up to 4 hours.

If your relief is not sufficient try a stronger concentration capsaicin cream, which comes in several strengths.

You won't develop a tolerance to it so you can use it night and day. Carry a tube of capsaicin cream with you everywhere and apply it when your pain reminds you. When puzzled friends see you frantically fumbling in your crotch, just say brightly, "I'm applying capsaicin to my inguinal region". They'll never ask again.

Acupuncture

Find a Chinese acupuncturist – they usually have offices in Chinese herb shops – show him the illustrations in these pages and describe your symptoms. Acupuncture can provide remarkable relief and should be included in everyone's regimen. Ignore the nonsense about acupuncture being painful. The little pinpricks are nothing compared to what you're suffering! In fact, they'll probably feel good because they immediately move your stuck energy. Ask your Chinese Medicine practitioner if there is an herbal prescription that might help. Chinese herbs are inexpensive and very effective.

Pain Management

There are pain management clinics in every major city. Before you spend the money, consider learning some pain management tricks yourself by reading the chapter, below, on pain management.

Weight Loss

If you're over your optimum weight then change your diet and eating habits and get regular exercise. And any extra weight prevents, complicates or delays your recovery.

The quickest, easiest, safest way to shed pounds is a juice fast: fresh, organic, raw fruit and vegetable juices, diluted 50% with water, for 10–30 days. If you don't own a juicer and can't borrow one, buy a Panasonic centrifugal juicer. Quick and, most important, EASY TO CLEAN – the secret to successful juicing!

Massage

Massage from a knowledgeable masseuse can be remarkably effective. Before your session take time to show them the anatomy illustration of the LFCN, talk about the L2/L3 junction, and discuss your symptoms. A qualified Thai masseuse can do wonders to relieve your symptoms – or at least distract you.

Walking up Stairs

Avoid walking as much as possible. Above all, don't make my mistake: you're feeling pretty good. All the things you've been doing are paying off: you feel no pain! So you climb the stairs like a normal person, taking great delight in being able to push off the stairs with your bad leg. Big mistake. That night will be agonizing, possibly the worst night since your symptoms started. For some reason, pushing off like that, and lifting your whole body weight by extending the ball of your foot exacerbates the problem. Be warned!

If you have a question, have novel symptoms of MP, or find a treatment or exercise that provides relief, please let me know by emailing godfree@gmail.com. I'll update this book so that everyone can benefit from your discovery.

EXERCISES FOR MERALGIA

Here are some simple, gentle stretches that relieve Meralgia symptoms and shorten your recovery time significantly. Be patient. This is a slow, gentle approach and will take 1-2 weeks to begin to bear fruit.

One-Legged Balance

- Stand on right leg.
- Tail wags *just your sacrum* to the opposite (left) side.
- Lift your left leg 1 inch off the floor and balance while you inhale and exhale.
- Repeat on the opposite side.
- Do this 3 times each side.

One-Leg Knee Bends

- Stand with even weight on both feet.
- Bend one knee while keeping your toes on the ground and your hips level.
- Repeat on the opposite side.
- Do this 3 times each side.

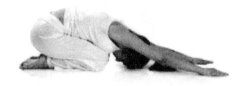

Child's Pose with Finger Walk
An enjoyable exercise to mobilize your
vertebrae:

- Kneel on the floor with your knees apart
  and your buttocks resting on your heels.

- Stretch out your arms in front of you with
  your fingers 'bridged' so that *only your
  finger tips* are touching the floor.

- Keeping your arms outstretched, *slowly*
  'walk' your fingers to the left as far as they
  will comfortably go, allowing your arms
  and torso to follow, but keeping your butt
  on your heels, while you inhale.

- Allow your torso and spine to bend gently
  to the left as your fingers do the walking.

- Pause, and then *slowly* 'walk' your fingers
  back to center as you exhale.

- Repeat the exercise to the right hand side,
  remembering to inhale and exhale fully.

- **Do this 3 times each side** every time you
  get out of bed, and at least 3 times every
  day.

Cat-Cow

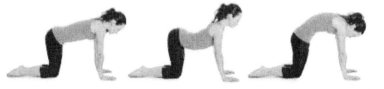

iStock

- Kneel on all fours on the floor.
- *Slowly* curl your tailbone down between your legs. As your tailbone is reaching its furthest limit, curl your head and neck down so that your back arches fully, like an angry cat's. Exhale slowly as you perform this exercise.
- Pause. Slowly uncurl neck and tailbone as you inhale. Allow your belly to drop *slowly*, like a cow's as your breath reaches its fullest point of inhalation.
- Do this 3 times each side.
- Repeat this cycle 3 times each day, with special attention to it as soon as you get up in the morning and just before you go to sleep.

The Half Bridge

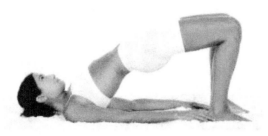

The woman in the picture is doing a full bridge. We don't need that much lift for our MP exercise, so we'll do a half bridge. Here's how

- Lie on your back with your knees bent and feet on the floor (the floor is best, but in bed is OK) and curl *just your tailbone* up very slowly, exhaling as you do so.

- Then slowly uncurl it and lay it flat again while inhaling.

- Bridge up and down focusing on how your L2-L3 joint is articulating: make your vertebrae move *individually*. It's slow work at first, but it feels good.

- Use your abs to slowly roll your vertebrae off the floor by curling your tailbone up, followed by each vertebra up only to T10.

- Then, just as slowly and carefully, roll your spine back down one vertebra at a time. **Do this 3 times.**

- Repeat the bridge imagining you have 3 spines instead of just one... and roll up the right side spine and then once you have reached the top of the bridge rotate through neutral to the left side and roll back down the left side spine.

- Switch directions and repeat
- Repeat, this time slowly curling your 5 lumbar vertebrae off the floor, one by one, while *exhaling*.
- Pause when you have curled all 5 up, and then uncurl as you inhale and lie flat.
- Pause; uncurl as slowly and deliberately as you came up, while *inhaling*.
- Repeat this exercise every 4 hours.

Note: *DO NOT* curl up as high as the lady in the photograph. She's demonstrating the "full bridge", which is not what we need right now.

One-Legged Bridge
As soon as you feel strong enough you can begin strengthening your affected leg by doing the one-legged bridge. Start small by bridging then lifting each foot an inch off the floor. As you grow stronger you can practice until you can do what the lady in the picture is doing.

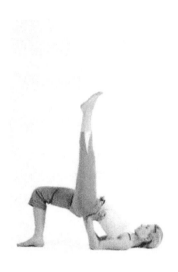

Note: **DO NOT** lift up as high as the lady in the photograph. She's demonstrating the full one-legged bridge, which is not what we need right now. Instead, try just lifting one foot just an inch off the ground, and then back down. Repeat on each side three times.

Theraband Leg and Thigh Exercises

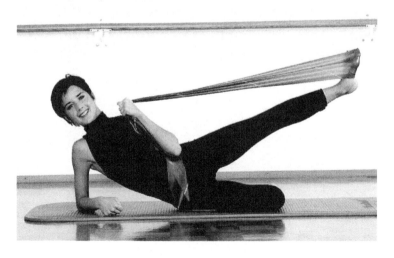

Therabands are stretchy bands that provide safe, passive resistance to your movements. You can buy them from Amazon or make your own by cutting up an old bicycle inner tube. Here are some easy Theraband exercises:

- Lie on your side with your knees drawn up and your thighs at 90 degrees to your torso.
- Wrap the Theraband loosely around both knees.
- Keep your lower knee and leg still while gently raising the upper knee. Hold, inhale and exhale, then lower your knee back down.
- Repeat on the opposite side.

When you're feeling stronger, try a variation of exercise while standing. Here's a video of the standing version, done with straight legs. You can play around with the Theraband; inventing exercises that will help bring your quads back into play and strengthen your hip/adductor muscles.

Quadriceps Stretches

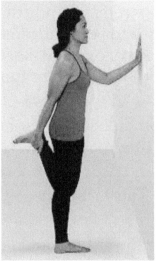

During a bout of meralgia our quads (and that whole side of the body) spend weeks or months contracted and unused. Now's the time to coad your muscle fibers back to their normal, healthy length and strength. Here are two variations of the same quadriceps stretch. The first, above, is easier. The second, below, allows you to work up to your pain/stretch threshold. It looks like this:

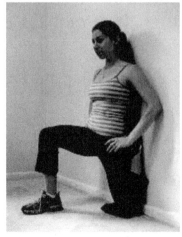

Foam Roller on Outer Quadriceps

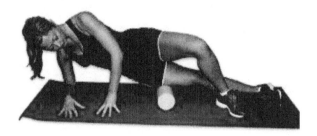

Foam rollers are cheap and effective tools for stretching muscles.

- Lie on one side supported by your elbow and, with the roller under your outer thigh, move slowly and gently up and down so that you "roll out" your contracted outer quadriceps.

- Repeat on the other leg so that you remain balanced, side to side.

Mobilizing the LFC Nerve Root Where it Exits Your Spine

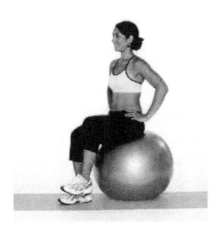

To recap: the lateral femoral cutaneous nerve is at the root of Meralgia Paraesthetica. The nerve root usually comes out of your spinal cord between the second lumbar vertebra, L2, and the third lumbar vertebra, L3. Mobilizing this L2–L3 region of your lumbar spine can provide real benefit:

Sit on a Geo Ball (from Amazon) with both feet planted and sitting tall through the chest, with a neutral, S-curve spine:

1. Rotate left – maintaining a neutral spine in terms of flexion or extension, then

2. Add a slow tail wag to you left from the bottom up.

3. Now you've got rotation/side bend. Now,

4. Add flexion by rolling the ball under you forward. and

5. Add extension by rolling the ball back.

6. Do this exercise first in rotation, then

7. Repeat it in side bend,

8. Repeat it in then flexion

9. Repeat it in extension

Do it in front of a mirror until you've gotten it down.

Repeat at least every morning and evening and...take your time. Enjoy the stretch! If my instructions are unclear schedule a session with a Physical Therapist, who should have Geo Balls, and ask her to guide you through it.

If you have a question, have novel symptoms of MP, or find a treatment or exercise that provides relief, please let me know by emailing godfree@gmail.com. I'll update this book so that everyone can benefit from your discovery.

WALKING AND SITTING

MP makes your simplest actions complicated and even painful. Here are some tips that will help:

1. Walk up stairs with your good leg. *Do not* push off with your painful leg.

- This means that you'll have both feet on each step before you lift your good leg up onto the next step and push up with that good leg.
- Allow the painful leg to follow passively.
- In other words, lead with your GOOD leg walking up stairs (even downstairs).

2. When going down stairs, lead with your 'bad' leg.

3. When climbing stairs, by habit you'll flex the ankle of your bad leg (whether going up or downstairs).

- DON'T FLEX YOUR ANKLE! At least not until you start to heal.
- Instead, move the foot of your bad leg consciously, keeping the foot level and the

ankle un-flexed. You will look like a total dork but it's worth it.

4. Walk as little as possible.

5. When you sit, sit on flat, level padded surfaces so that your feet are flat on the floor, your knees are bent at 90 degrees, your thighs are horizontal, and your calves are vertical

6. Avoid sitting in deep, low couches, or anywhere that your thighs are not perpendicular to your torso. Always sit with your knees directly above your ankles.

If you have a question, have novel symptoms of MP, or find a treatment or exercise that provides relief, please let me know by emailing godfree@gmail.com. I'll update this book so that everyone can benefit from your discovery.

HYPNOSIS FOR PAIN MANAGEMENT

How can hypnosis affect pain management? The results from three lines of research have combined to create a renewed interest in the application of hypnosis for chronic pain management.

First, imaging studies demonstrate that the effects of hypnotic suggestions on brain activity are real and can target specific aspects of pain. Hypnosis for decreases in the intensity of pain result not only in significant decreases in pain intensity, but also decreases in activity in the brain areas that underlie the experience of pain intensity. At the same time, hypnotic suggestions for decrease in the unpleasantness (but not intensity) of pain have significant effects on how bad the pain makes people feel, but not necessarily intensity. Interestingly, these suggestions result in decreases in activity in the areas of the brain responsible for processing the emotional aspect of pain, but not those areas that are responsible for processing pain intensity.

Second, research studies demonstrate that hypnotic treatments can save money.

Hypnotic suggestions for reduced pain and improved healing have been shown to reduce the time needed for medical procedures, speed recovery time, and result in fewer analgesics needed — all of which not only result in more comfort for the patient, but save the patient and the patient's insurance companies money. In a time of growing medical expenses, it's nice to have a treatment that can actually result in cost savings.

Third, a rapidly growing body of research shows that hypnosis works. When hypnosis and hypnotic suggestions are combined with other treatments, those other treatments become more effective. When people with chronic pain are taught how to use self-hypnosis for pain management and improved sleep, they experience pain relief and sleep better. This research also reveals that hypnosis has many "side effects", which are overwhelmingly positive. People who learn self-hypnosis can not only experience significant pain relief, but report a greater sense of overall well-being and control.

For all of these reasons, more clinicians are seeking to learn how to apply hypnosis and to teach self-hypnosis to their clients with chronic pain. – From *Hypnosis for Chronic Pain Management* by Mark P. Jensen, Professor and Vice

Chair for Research of the Department of Rehabilitation Medicine at the University of Washington Medical Center.

As Dr. Jensen points out, hypnotherapy is safe, cheap and quick. I've seen its effectiveness and feel it is worth trying. A *caveat*: many hypnotherapists want to spend one or more visits "evaluating" you. While understandable, this process is frustrating and expensive. When making an appointment with a hypnotherapist ask if they will treat you on your first visit. If they seem reluctant, ask what information they need you to send them so that you can email it to them in advance.

I asked Dr. Jensen if he had experience with meralgia paresthetica and hypnosis. Here's his reply:

Dear Dr. Roberts,

I am not aware of any research performed here that has studied meralgia paresthetica, specifically. My work has focused on psychosocial treatments (e.g., CBT, hypnosis, neurofeedback) for chronic pain problems in general, including both neuropathic and nonneuropathic pain.

We have found that hypnosis is effective for reducing pain (but rarely "cures" pain -

- individuals should continue to practice to maintain "lower" levels of pain) for every type of pain problem we have used it with ON AVERAGE. However, some people respond very very well, and others not so much. Treatment response is variable. In general, I have noticed it is more effective for neuropathic pain than non-neuropathic pain, but I have not directly compared central neuropathic pain to peripheral neuropathic pain (MP is a peripheral problem). It is possible that hypnosis is more effective for central neuropathic pain problems than all other pain problems (including non-neuropathic pain and peripheral neuropathic pain).

That said, if I have a loved one with MP, I would definitely recommend that they see a qualified (careful, there are many nonqualified practitioners of hypnosis) practitioner and learn self-hypnosis skills.

Hope this helps! Cheers,

Mark

Mark P. Jensen, Ph.D., Professor and Vice Chair for Research, Department of Rehabilitation Medicine, University of Washington

If you have a question, have novel symptoms of MP, or find a treatment or exercise that provides relief, please let me know by emailing godfree@gmail.com. I'll update this book so that everyone can benefit from your discovery.

HOW DOCTORS VIEW MERALGIA

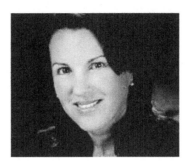

Orly Avitzur, Yale University MD Neurologist answers doctors' questions about Meralgia:

What treatment modes are available for Meralgia paresthetica (MP)? How often is surgical decompression needed? If required, what would be the indications and who is the best person to do it -- a general surgeon, a neurosurgeon, or some other specialist? Can injection of lidocaine at the start of the nerve's course in the thigh be helpful?

MP is a condition characterized by numbness, tingling, pain, irritation, or burning in the anterior or anterolateral thigh resulting from compression or injury to the lateral femoral cutaneous nerve. Causes include mechanical factors, such as compressive clothing, belts, obesity, and pregnancy. MP has also reportedly occurred following surgical procedures and trauma, or has been related to plexopathy due to mass or hemorrhage. A recent study found that the incidence rate of MP is 4.3/10,000 persons per year and that it is found in higher numbers in patients suffering from carpal tunnel syndrome (suggesting a predisposition to nerve entrapment syndromes) and during pregnancy.

Successful treatment can often be achieved with conservative therapy, such as physical therapy, acupuncture, weight reduction to shrink abdominal girth, avoiding constrictive garments, and using analgesics and other medications.

Medications used in other forms of neuropathic pain, such as tricyclic antidepressants or anticonvulsants, may alleviate some of the symptoms of pain, dysesthesias, or paresthesias. The advent of the newer antiepileptic drugs with weight-reducing effects may be ideally suited to those patients in whom obesity is a factor, and diet and weight loss are goals.

Injection of a local anesthetic may be helpful in establishing the diagnosis but only gives temporary relief. If successful, local blocks with steroids may be effective. A report from a pain clinic found that a treatment plan of repeated, subsequent injection blocks on alternate days was successful. They used .25% of bupivacaine combined with methylprednisolone acetate in divided doses of 20 mg each, up to a maximum of 80-120 mg along with oral diphenylhydantoin (100-300 mg daily), and 85% of their population attained complete relief within 10 weeks.

Surgery is generally reserved for patients with persistent and debilitating pain refractory to other modalities of treatment. Various techniques have been used, and it is not clear whether neurolysis or transaction is the procedure of choice; some believe that the best results may be achieved by local decompression in combination with neurolysis via the infrainguinal ligament approach. Surgery is most often performed by neurosurgeons, but general surgeons or orthopaedists may be involved, depending on the institution.

References

1 van Slobbe AM, Bohnen AM, Bernsen RM, et al. Incidence rates and determinants in Meralgia paresthetica in general practice. J Neurol. 2004;25:294-297.

2 Aigner N, Aigner G, Fialka C, Fritz A. Therapy of Meralgia paresthetica with acupuncture. Two case reports. Schmerz. 1997;11:113-115.

3 Dureja GP, Gulaya V, Jayalakshmi TS, Mandal P. Management of Meralgia paresthetica: a multimodality regimen. Anesth Analg. 1995;80:1060-1061. Abstract

4 Mirzai S, Penkert G, Samii M. Long term results of surgical treatment in patients with Meralgia paresthetica. Clin Neur Neurosurg. 1997:99:S120.

– With thanks to <u>Medscape</u>.

If you have a question, have novel symptoms of MP, or find a treatment or exercise that provides relief, please let me know by emailing godfree@gmail.com. I'll update this book so that everyone can benefit from your discovery.

PREGNANCY AND CAT-COW

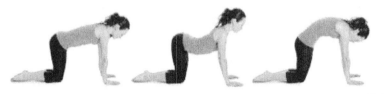

iStock

Tight clothing, obesity or weight gain, and pregnancy are common causes of Meralgia paresthetica. Since all four often occur together, it is not surprising that MP regularly afflicts pregnant women. The good news is that pregnant women are usually young and otherwise healthy so recovery should be rapid once you correct the underlying causes. You can find fast-acting, natural measures throughout this book. One yoga exercise that is particularly effective for pregnant women is Cat-Cow, which looks (above) like it sounds. Performed slowly, timed to the in-breath (cow) and out-breath (cat), it is extremely enjoyable and relaxing. The "cat" posture is best generated by tucking your tailbone steadily down, allowing that movement to raise your spine in a gentle arch. ***Here's a video of Cat Cow in action***.

If you have a question, have novel symptoms of MP, or find a treatment or exercise that provides relief, please let me know by emailing godfree@gmail.com. I'll update this book so that everyone can benefit from your discovery.

SURGERY ON 7
PATIENTS

Fifteen cases of meralgia paresthetica were
identified in 14 patients. The LFCN was affected
unilaterally in 13 patients and bilaterally in 1
patient. Involvement of the LFCN was
confirmed in each instance by injecting a small
amount of bupivacaine with epinephrine around
the LFCN where it passed near the anterior
superior iliac spine. The accuracy of the
injection was confirmed by obtaining
anterolateral thigh paresthesia, and in each case
the symptoms were completely relieved for
several hours.

On follow-up visits, the patients were given a
second injection in the same area using a
mixture of bupivacaine and methylprednisolone,
and they again obtained complete relief. Five
patients had no further symptoms in follow-up
ranging from 28 to 60 months. Nine patients
had recurrence of their symptoms 2 to 4 weeks
after the second injection. These patients were
typically injected a third time to ensure that the
results were reproducible. These patients also
underwent computed tomography or magnetic
resonance imaging examinations of the lower
back and pelvis to rule out discogenic disease or
other pathology.

Seven patients in this group subsequently opted for surgical treatment of their meralgia paresthetica.

Results of Surgery
Between 1992 and 1996, four women and three men underwent surgery for meralgia paresthetica. **Symptoms had been present from 2 to 15 years. Three of the patients had a total of five previous operations performed elsewhere, but none of the operations resulted in relief**. These operations included femoral head core decompression, groin exploration, iliotibial Z-plasty, and ilioinguinal nerve resection.

Patients frequently could not stand to wear tight clothing or carry keys in the pocket of the affected side. One patient with an above-knee amputation could not wear his prosthesis because of the thigh dysesthesia. In addition, three patients also had lower lateral leg pain on the affected side (Fig. 1C). This lower leg pain was perceived by the patients as being related to but distinct from the thigh dysesthesias. **All of these symptoms were relieved after resection** (surgical removal of all or part of of the LFCN).

Considering the preceding reports as well as observations from the present series, it appears that meralgia paresthetica patients who have failed to respond to conservative management can be considered in three subsets:

- Adults with less than 1 year of symptoms and all pediatric patients should undergo simple decompression.
- Patients in the first group who have persistent or recurrent symptoms should be considered for resection.
- Adult patients with symptoms present more than 1 year should be considered for primary resection.

When resection is indicated, the LFCN should be divided several centimeters posterior to the anterior superior iliac spine. This has the advantage of avoiding any scar tissue from previous decompression surgery and provides a single larger nerve for dissection. In addition, this places the transected nerve trunk in a protected area that is not likely to be stimulated. In my experience the anesthetic area created by resection is well tolerated and tends to shrink during several months.

Conclusions
Meralgia paresthetica remains an obscure diagnosis for many physicians and is frequently overlooked or misdiagnosed. Many of the previous authors have not had the benefit of magnetic resonance imaging or computed tomography, and it is likely that some of the patients reported in the earlier series were

actually suffering from discogenic disease or other disorders of the central nervous system. The confusion in diagnosis by some of the earlier authors, plus the fact that many of these authors reported results with very brief follow-up, probably accounts for some of the disagreement concerning the treatment of meralgia paresthetica.

Despite this, meralgia paresthetica is not rare, it is readily recognized, and it responds favorably to adequate treatment. Read more...
– Gregory K. Ivins, MD, FACS.

*If you have a question, have novel symptoms of MP, or find a treatment or exercise that provides relief, please let me know by emailing godfree@gmail.com.
I'll update this book so that everyone can benefit from your discovery.*

PAIN MANAGEMENT

This section includes brief summaries of previous chapters along with other therapies that are gradually being included in this emerging field of practice. Pain management, or *pain medicine*, draws on science and the healing arts to systematically study pain, its evaluation, prevention, diagnosis and treatment, and rehabilitation. An excellent textbook is Bonica's Management of Pain. Buy a used copy at Amazon ($20) and educate yourself.

Pain management is usually distinguished from surgical treatment and the techniques it uses may be employed
- To identify the source of a patient's pain
- As part of an aggressive-conservative, nonsurgical care program
- To help determine the areas to be addressed surgically
- To help rehabilitate patients after surgery
- For patients after surgery to cope with residual or recalcitrant pain

Pain management uses a wide variety of techniques to address pain and painful disorders, some of which have no experimental support and some whose effectiveness has been demonstrated in clinical trials. Here's a brief overview:

Pain Management Techniques

Pain management techniques can be grouped in terms of their invasiveness.

- Some, like physical therapy, are non-invasive and don't involve the use of medications
- Some, such as pain medications, are purely pharmacologic in nature
- Some involve invasive techniques like injections

Noninvasive Non-Drug Pain Management

There's a wide variety of non-invasive, non-drug pain management techniques. Here are a few:

- **Exercise** - physical exertion with the aim of increasing strength, increasing flexibility, and restoring normal motion. Includes the McKenzie method, water therapy, stretching exercises, aerobic routines and many others. May involve active, passive and resistive elements. Exercise is necessary for proper cardiovascular health, disc nutrition and musculoskeletal health.
- **Manual techniques** - manipulation of affected areas by applying force to the joints, muscles, and ligaments. Some evidence for the effectiveness of certain techniques is available.

- **Behavioral modification** - use of behavioral methods to optimize patient responses to back pain and painful stimuli. Cognitive therapy involves teaching the patient to alleviate back pain by means of relaxation techniques, coping techniques and other methods. Biofeedback involves learning to control muscle tension, blood pressure, and heart rate for symptomatic improvement.
- **Superficial heating or cooling of skin** - These pain management methods include cold packs and hot packs, ultrasound, and diathermy and should be used in conjunction with exercise.
- **Electrotherapy** - the most commonly known form of electrotherapy is transcutaneous electrical nerve stimulation (TENS). TENS therapy attempts to reduce pain by means of a low-voltage electric stimulation that interacts with the sensory nervous system. Randomized controlled trials have yielded either positive or neutral results regarding the efficacy of TENS as a treatment for back pain.

Noninvasive Pharmacologic Pain Management

Pain relievers and related drugs are used at every stage of the medical treatment of pain, from the initial onset of acute pain to facilitation of rehabilitation, treatment of chronic pain and alleviation of pain in cases of failed surgery. The most common noninvasive pharmacologic treatments for chronic back pain are:

- **Analgesics** - or pain medications, including acetaminophen. Long-term use may involve risk of kidney or liver damage.
- **Nonsteroidal anti-inflammatory agents (NSAIDs)** - includes aspirin, ibuprofen, naproxen and COX-2 inhibitors. Long-term use may cause gastrointestinal ulcers, and may slightly raise the risk of heart attack.
- **Muscle relaxants** - used to treat muscle spasms due to pain and protective mechanisms.
- **Narcotic medications** - most appropriate for acute or post-operative pain. Since use of narcotics entails risk of habituation or addiction if not properly supervised, they are not often used for chronic conditions.
- **Antidepressants and anticonvulsants** - used to treat neuropathic ("nerve") pain.
- **Neuromodulating medications** - used to treat neuropathic and muscular pain.

Invasive Pain Management Techniques

Invasive techniques in pain management involve injections and/or placement of devices into the body. The most popular invasive pain management techniques include:

- **Injections (also known as blocks)**
- Injections provide direct delivery of steroids or anesthetic into joints, ligaments, muscles, or around nerves. These injections may provide relief of pain (often temporary) and can be used to confirm if the injected structure is the source of the pain, clarifying the diagnosis. Epidural injections can provide temporary relief for upper extremity or lower extremity pain due to a pinched nerve in the spine.
- **Prolotherapy.** This technique involves injection of an irritant solution to stimulate blood circulation and ligament repair at affected site. The effectiveness of this technique is not known.
- **Radiofrequency radioablation.** This involves deadening of painful nerves via heat administered through a small needle. In carefully selected patients, this helps in approximately 60% of patients and lasts for months to years.
- **Surgically implanted electrotherapy devices.** These are implantable spinal cord stimulators (SCS) and implantable peripheral nerve stimulators.

- **Implantable opioid infusion pumps.**
  These surgically implanted pumps deliver
  opioids directly to the spinal cord. The
  pumps are expensive and their
  effectiveness is controversial.

Pain Management Specialists

There is no single field of medicine or health
care that is the preferred approach to pain
management. The premise of pain management
is that it's essential to take a
multidisciplinary approach. so pain
management specialists are most commonly
found in:

- Physical medicine and rehabilitation.
  (*Physiatry*)
- Anesthesiology
- Interventional radiology
- Physical therapy
- Specialists in psychology, psychiatry,
  behavioral science and other areas who
  may also play an important role in a
  comprehensive pain management
  program.

Most pain management specialists are referred
through a physician. Talk to yours about a pain
management program. Keep in mind that there
are many varieties of pain management
programs to explore, which makes it confusing
and frustrating at times so it's important point is
to work proactively with your health
professionals and not to give up if you don't

initially succeed. This process is challenging when you're enduring intense pain but once you find an approach that you're comfortable with your condition and pain levels should improve.

Managing Chronic Pain

The first step is to receive a thorough medical evaluation to determine its cause.

- In some situations, such as a herniated disc in the spine, it may be important to pay attention to the level and type of pain so that it can serve as a warning signal of impending damage.
- In other cases, especially when the pain is chronic and the health condition is unchangeable, one goal can be to try and keep the chronic pain from being the entire focus of your life.

Whatever your medical condition, there are a number of effective strategies for coping with chronic back pain, including:

- **Relaxation training**: Relaxation involves concentration and slow, deep breathing to release tension from muscles and relieve pain. Learning to relax takes practice, but relaxation training focuses attention away from pain and releases tension from all muscles. Relaxation apps are widely available to help you learn these skills and I've listed some in the Resources page at the end of this book.

- **Biofeedback**: Biofeedback is taught by professionals using special machines to help you learn to control bodily functions like heart rate and muscle tension. As you learn to release muscle tension, the machine immediately indicates success. Once you master it you can practice it without the machine.
- **Visual imagery** and distraction: involves concentrating on mental pictures of pleasant scenes or events or mentally repeating positive words or phrases to reduce pain. Recordings and apps are available to help you learn visual imagery skills.
- **Distraction techniques** focus your attention away from negative or painful images to positive mental thoughts. From watching TV or a movie, reading a book or listening to a book on tape, listening to music, or talking to a friend.
- **Hypnosis**: Some people are hypnotized by a therapist and given a post-hypnotic suggestion that reduces the pain they feel. Others are taught self-hypnosis and can hypnotize themselves when pain interrupts their ability to function. Self-hypnosis is a form of relaxation training.

RECOVERING FROM MP

If you neglect the rehabilitation step, Meralgia can leave you permanently impaired--most commonly with a permanently weak, flaccid or shrunken leg and a permanent limp.

Factors which influence the speed of your recovery include
1. Your age
2. The duration of your MP affliction
3. The severity of your case
4. How diligently you work on rehabilitation. As you can see, this is the only factor you control.

As a general rule, allow at least *six weeks of ACTIVE rehab work for every week you spent in bed.* If you were in bed for a month, look forward to 6 months of twice-daily exercises. If you've been following the advice in these pages you'll notice your symptoms diminishing in 4–6 weeks. Here are some ways to make exercise easy and effective:

1. TAKE A BEGINNERS' YOGA CLASS.
Why? Because you've been lying down for weeks and your body has been knotted with pain. Gentle stretching will un-knot it and relax your leg dramatically, making you much easier to be

around: your grumpiness will decline dramatically. Explain your situation to the yoga teacher before class begins. She'll encourage you to take it easy, and so you should. You'll be surprised how quickly the 90 minutes flies by. And how good you feel afterwards.

2. QUIT THE DRUGS ONE AT A TIME.
Your withdrawal headaches will be mild this way. Quit the GABA drugs last. Their euphoria will make the withdrawal from other drugs more tolerable.

3. SAVE NORMAL STAIR-CLIMBING UNTIL LAST.
Pushing off with your 'bad' leg can make your symptoms flare up. Start by walking normally up or down one (preferably low) stair. Next day, make it two. Etc.

4. WEAK LEG SYNDROME
Weak Leg Syndrome (WLS) is a name I made up to remind you that, for weeks or months (or, in my case, years) after you get out of bed, your 'bad' leg will be untrustworthy. It will be weak and wobbly, and prone to collapse without warning if you put too much weight on it. It's annoying because you will be able to walk normally and you will look normal, but your leg will betray you just when you least expect it.

Instead of the sympathy your groans elicited while you were in agony, now people will think you're drunk or feeble as you lurch around or collapse pathetically on the ground. Be of good cheer. This is part of recuperation. You are actually getting better and one day--usually in a few months--this, too, shall pass!

My 12-Month Recovery From MP

It's now 12 months since I contracted Meralgia paresthetica. I'm 73 years old, and my recovery is probably slower because of my age. Here's what I've learned so far:

You can contract Meralgia paresthetica from being too skinny, just as you can from being too fat. I'm naturally slim and last summer I lost my fat layer during a long, hot, tropical summer. Then I did a yoga pose, a seated forward bend called Janu Sirsasana (pictured) with my foot tucked into my groin before bending forward. When I bent over to touch my head on my knee, the blade of my foot crushed my lateral femoral cutaneous nerve and presto! Meralgia paresthetica. Six painful weeks in bed and 12 months of slow recovery.

Recovery is very, very slow. I was able to begin yoga again –t he best cure, paradoxically, because it stretches all the muscles – after 9 months. At first I was only strong enough to attend one class each week. All during that time I was still favoring my injured leg and clinging to the handrail every time I used the stairs. Only after 12 months was I able to resume three classes a week. Now my leg is getting noticeably stronger every week. But it has still lost muscle mass and muscle tone due to contraction and non-use. And my core (abdominal) strength is still far below where it was before I got MP.

I'll write more as I pass various milestones on the way to full recovery. I'd like to hear from anyone else who's recuperating from MP, of course. Email me at the address on the bottom of the page. I'll instantly update this book so that others can benefit from your discovery.

If you have a question, have novel symptoms of MP, or find a treatment or exercise that provides relief, please let me know by emailing godfree@gmail.com. I'll update this book so that everyone can benefit from your discovery.

CLAIMING DISABILITY FOR MERALGIA

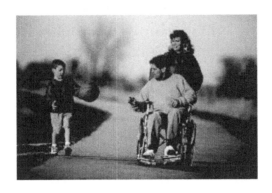

If you need to claim disability insurance you should know what your doctor – or your insurance company's doctor – uses when she fills out their forms. Here are the Medical Disability Guidelines which all doctors consult for disability cases:

Meralgia paresthetica ("thigh pain and paresthesia") is a condition in which a sensory nerve (the lateral femoral cutaneous nerve) in the front and outer (anterolateral) thigh becomes compressed, resulting in symptoms of pain, as well as tingling and numbness (paresthesia). It is caused by entrapment of the lateral femoral cutaneous nerve, which originates at the second and third lumbar nerve roots and ends at the anterolateral thigh. The nerve can become entrapped anywhere along its course, but is most frequently compressed where it exits the pelvis and enters the thigh beneath the inguinal ligament at the front of the hip. It also can be compressed adjacent to the spine or within the abdominal cavity. The nerve may be compressed externally from restrictive seatbelts or tight clothing (e.g., belts, trousers) or internally from the pressure of pregnancy, a pelvic tumor, or abscess. The lateral femoral cutaneous nerve also may become injured from direct trauma to the hip and thigh or during surgery (e.g., replacement, appendectomy, hysterectomy).

Meralgia paresthetica typically is unilateral, although it may present bilaterally in up to 20% of cases (Luzzio; Sekul).

Risk

Meralgia paresthetica is most common in individuals between the ages of 30 and 65 (Kornbluth). Individuals with mellitus, thyroid, and alcoholism are at increased risk for developing peripheral neuropathies, including Meralgia paresthetica. Meralgia paresthetica is slightly more common in males than females (Luzzio), especially in those who must wear tight belts (e.g., policemen with duty belts, carpenters with tool belts, soldiers with body armor) (Sekul).

Obese individuals are at increased risk for developing Meralgia paresthetica from restrictive clothing, but thinner individuals undergoing spinal surgery have a higher risk of developing the disorder from inadequately padded positioning on the surgical table. Meralgia paresthetica is a complication of spinal surgery in 12% to 20% of cases (Benzel).

Incidence and Prevalence
Meralgia paresthetica is thought to be present in 7% to 35% of individuals with complaints of leg pain (Luzzio). Prevalence of Meralgia paresthetica is 30 individuals per 100,000 population (Kornbluth). Incidence of Meralgia paresthetica is 43 cases per 100,000 person-years (Sekul).

Diagnosis

History: The individual may describe altered sensations in the anterolateral thigh, which may include sharp or dull pain, burning, aching, tingling, hypersensitivity, or numbness. In most cases, the individual will report a slow (insidious) onset of symptoms, although pain may occur suddenly from direct trauma to the hip or thigh or following a long car or plane journey. Typically, symptoms will not extend below the knee and may be worse after prolonged sitting, standing, squatting, or when moving from sit to stand. Individuals also may report increased symptoms after sleeping in prolonged prone or fetal positions in which the hip is at end range flexion or extension.
Physical exam: Because the lateral femoral cutaneous nerve is purely sensory, muscle

strength and deep tendon reflexes should remain normal. There should be no observable muscle atrophy. Light touch and pinprick testing may reveal a large patch of reduced sensation at the anterolateral thigh. Movement of the affected limb into hip extension may increase symptoms, as the position may increase tension on the lateral femoral cutaneous nerve. Firmly touching the front of the hip (deep palpation) may reproduce painful symptoms (pelvic compression test); this test has a sensitivity of 95% and specificity of 93.3% for the condition (Nouraei). Direct tapping by the examiner over the nerve as it passes beneath the inguinal ligament at the anterior hip may reproduce painful symptoms (Tinel sign). A full neurological examination should be performed to rule out spinal origins of thigh pain.

Tests: Laboratory blood tests may include complete blood count (CBC), uric acid, erythrocyte sedimentation rate (ESR), antinuclear antibodies (ANA), and tests to help rule out underlying thyroid disorders, diabetes, and other metabolic diseases. Imaging studies generally are not useful in diagnosing this disorder, although x-rays may help rule out lumbar origins of thigh pain. In some cases, electromyography (EMG) and nerve conduction studies may be ordered to confirm the diagnosis, establish the severity of nerve compression, and rule out lumbar radiculopathy.

Treatment

Meralgia paresthetica is treated conservatively by identifying and alleviating the point(s) of compression of the lateral femoral cutaneous nerve. Patient education to modify aggravating activities and discontinue wearing compressive items of clothing is indicated to relieve nerve compression.

Stretching of tight structures (e.g., hip flexors, quadriceps muscles) overlying the nerve may be helpful. If the individual is obese, counseling to reduce body weight should be included.

If symptoms persist after lifestyle modification, conservative management with over-the-counter nonsteroidal anti-inflammatory drugs (NSAIDs) and local pain-relieving modalities such as lidocaine patches or corticosteroid injection may be necessary. In some cases, anticonvulsant medications or tricyclic antidepressants may give relief of symptoms.

Rarely, surgery may be needed to release the nerve (neurolysis) or move the nerve to a location of less compression (transposition).

Practice Guidelines

The American College Occupational and Environmental Medicine's Practice Guidelines, the gold standard in effective medical treatment of occupational injuries and illnesses, are provided in this section to complement the disability duration guidelines. Some of this is a repeat of what's above, but there is some interesting additional information that could be useful to anyone with MP.

Prognosis

In most cases, once the source of nerve compression is identified and eliminated, the symptoms fully resolve and the nerve heals; in mild cases, resolution of symptoms may occur within hours or weeks (Craig). If nerve compression is caused by pregnancy, the condition is alleviated following childbirth. Many times, the condition is self-limited and may heal spontaneously.

Rehabilitation

The focus of rehabilitation for Meralgia paresthetica is to alleviate symptoms while modifying activities to allow nerve healing. Heat or ice may be used to relieve pain. Electrical stimulation, transcutaneous electrical nerve stimulation (TENS), and ultrasound also may be helpful to reduce symptoms and facilitate muscle relaxation before stretching (Craig; Luzzio).

Stretching exercises and trigger point therapy may be indicated to reduce tightness of hip and thigh muscles (e.g., hip flexors, quadriceps) that may contribute to the nerve compression.

An important component of physical therapy is instructing the individual in postural education and lifestyle modification to avoid sitting with the legs crossed, prolonged sitting or standing, or other postures in which the nerve may become compressed. Because it is important to

eliminate all causes of nerve compression, individuals are instructed to wear loose clothing and to initiate a weight loss regimen and general conditioning program (Craig).
A home exercise program should be taught to complement supervised rehabilitation and to be continued after the completion of physical therapy.

Complications

Complications of unresolved Meralgia paresthetica include chronic pain and permanent tingling or numbness of the anterolateral thigh. Conservative management of the condition is successful in up to 91% of cases (Kornbluth). Surgery to release the nerve (neurolysis) is successful in resolving symptoms in 30% to 50% of cases, whereas cutting the nerve (transection) is successful in 82% of cases (Kornbluth). However, following lateral femoral cutaneous nerve transection, there will be permanent numbness of the anterolateral thigh.

Return to Work (Restrictions/Accommodations)

Modifications to the work environment may be necessary to limit prolonged standing and walking, as well as prolonged sitting. If the individual is required to travel for work, modifications to the travel schedule may be needed during recovery. Additional time off to attend rehabilitation sessions may be required. If pain medication is needed after return to work, company policy on its use should be reviewed to determine if medication usage is compatible with job safety and function.

Regarding Diagnosis

- Did individual report sharp or dull pain, burning, aching, tingling, hypersensitivity, or numbness anterolateral thigh?

- Did symptoms begin slowly (insidious onset), or quickly following direct trauma to the hip or thigh or following a long car or plane journey?

- Were symptoms limited to the thigh, not extending below the knee?

- Did individual report worsening of symptoms after prolonged sitting, standing, squatting, or when moving from sit to stand? After sleeping in prolonged prone or fetal positions?

- Did light touch and pinprick testing reveal a large patch of reduced sensation at the anterolateral thigh?

- Was individual's muscle strength and deep tendon reflexes normal?

- Did movement of the affected limb into hip extension increase symptoms?

- Did firmly touching the front of the hip (deep palpation) reproduce painful symptoms (pelvic compression test)?
- Was Tinel sign present over the anterior hip?
- Did laboratory blood tests reveal underlying thyroid disorders, diabetes, and other metabolic diseases? Is individual an alcoholic? Obese?
- Were EMG and nerve conduction studies necessary to confirm the diagnosis?
- Was diagnosis of Meralgia paresthetica confirmed?

Regarding Treatment

- Were points of nerve compression identified and eliminated with lifestyle modification and avoidance of wearing compressive items of clothing? Did this resolve symptoms?
- Is individual stretching tight structures (e.g., hip flexors, quadriceps muscles) overlying the nerve? Has this been helpful?
- Is physical therapy indicated? Is individual compliant with home exercise program for stretching? Has individual initiated a general conditioning program?
- If individual is obese, is s/he receiving counseling to reduce body weight?

- If symptoms did not resolve with lifestyle modification, is conservative management with NSAIDs indicated?
- Are anticonvulsant medications or tricyclic antidepressants necessary?
- Has individual received local pain-relieving modalities such as lidocaine patches or corticosteroid injection? Was this helpful?
- Was surgery necessary for severe, prolonged symptoms to release the nerve (neurolysis) or move the nerve to a location of less compression (transposition)?

Regarding Prognosis

- Did adequate time elapse for full recovery?
- Were modifications made to the individual's job requirements during recovery?
- Has physical therapy been completed as recommended? Would additional therapy benefit individual?
- If lidocaine patches, corticosteroid injection, or surgery were necessary, did symptoms resolve?
- Does individual have any comorbid conditions that may interfere with a full

recovery?

— Medical Disability Advisor

If you have a question, have novel symptoms of MP, or find a treatment or exercise that provides relief, please let me know by emailing godfree@gmail.com.
I'll update this book so that everyone can benefit from your discovery.

MERALGIA SUFFERERS' REPORTS

Hi – about 2 months ago I suddenly got (what I now know is) Meralgia Parathesia in my right thigh following a slight back issue. Was in excruciating pain in spite of a series of ever increasing strength painkillers prescribed by GP who was not a great deal of help. Passed out with pain twice & ended up in hopsital for a day. Physio was ok but recovery progress was slow & improvement seemed to have stalled after 3 weeks – not good for the mind! So decided to trawl internet & eventually found this website that is so informative. The self help page with the 3 exercises was just what I was looking for. Have been doing the exercises for 2 weeks now & improvement has been amazing & I am almost back to normal. I can't thank you enough as it felt pretty bleak until I found out what I should be doing via your website. Pity my GP hasn't had a look !! – **David Brown**

I have been suffering severe Meralgia Paresthetica for almost six years now, each year the pain has gotten progressively worse, therefore my quality of life has decreased as I try to get through the day... And the night. I was super fit, had my personal training *business, ran and stretched every day, ate healthy and didn't abuse my body. I began to suffer during my third pregnancy, my OBGYN did not diagnose, I made the self diagnose through many days at google sites.. Then someone did listen to me, got tested, I've tried Garbepenten in combination with Endep, and made absolutely no difference, I had a couple anaesthetic blocks, which also have not had any effect...I have problems walking, cannot bear anyone touching my leg, cannot sit my children on my lap, can't bear the thought of going to the beach as the last time , the waves really hurt me badly. Even the simplest of stretches are a distant memory, now I can't even do a quad stretch. My neurologist has tried to talk me into having surgery but with such a low success rate and a very high chance that it may come back worse I have not given in to his recommendations. Feel very frustrated and a distant person of who I really want to be...*__Mexnzaus__

RESOURCES

Relaxation Apps

Some of these tracks are really, really cool.
Offbeat, even exotic and strange, but
compelling. Just right for sleepless nights.

itunes

- Relaxing Melodies

- Advanced Binaural Relaxation

- Best Relaxation Music

- More Relaxation Music

- Ambiance

- Qi Gong Music

- Buddha Machine

Android

- White Noise Lite
- Relax Completely

- Relaxing Sounds
- Music Therapy for Refreshment
- Calming Music to Tranquilize

- Relax & Sleep
- Relax Melodies
- Qi Gong Meditation Relaxation
- Buddhist Meditation Trainer

The National Institutes of Health Database

The National Institutes of Health, a national treasure, contains over 200 articles on Meralgia Paresthetica. Browse them to your heart's content. Here is the first page:

Select item 31989721.
Meralgia paresthetica: Relation to obesity, advanced age, and diabetes mellitus
Thomas J. Parisi, Jay Mandrekar, P. James B. Dyck, Christopher J. Klein
Neurology. 2011 October 18; 77(16): 1538–1542. doi: 10.1212/WNL.0b013e318233b356
PMCID:
PMC3198972
ArticlePubReaderPDF–549K

Select item 31940322.
Meralgia Paresthetica and Femoral Acetabular Impingement: A Possible Association
Aiesha Ahmed
J Clin Med Res. 2010 December; 2(6): 274–276. Published online 2010 December 11. doi: 10.4021/jocmr468w
PMCID:
PMC3194032
ArticlePubReaderPDF–182K

Select item 33158613.
Chiropractic management of chronic idiopathic **meralgia** paresthetica: a case study
Sébastien Houle
J Chiropr Med. 2012 March; 11(1): 36–41.
doi: 10.1016/j.jcm.2011.06.008

PMCID:
PMC3315861
ArticlePubReaderPDF–530K

Select item 31115604.
Ultrasound-guided Lateral Femoral Cutaneous Nerve Block in **Meralgia** Paresthetica
Jeong Eun Kim, Sang Gon Lee, Eun Ju Kim, Byung Woo Min, Jong Suk Ban, Ji Hyang Lee
Korean J Pain. 2011 June; 24(2): 115–118.
Published online 2011 June 3. doi: 10.3344/kjp.2011.24.2.115

PMCID:
PMC3111560
ArticlePubReaderPDF–640K

Select item 32062815.
Pulsed Radiofrequency Neuromodulation Treatment on the Lateral Femoral Cutaneous Nerve for the Treatment of**Meralgia** Paresthetica

Hyuk Jai Choi, Seok Keun Choi, Tae Sung Kim, Young Jin Lim
J Korean Neurosurg Soc. 2011 August; 50(2): 151–153. Published online 2011 August 31. doi: 10.3340/jkns.2011.50.2.151
PMCID:
PMC3206281
ArticlePubReaderPDF–748K

Select item 30300656.
Meralgia paresthetica affecting parturient women who underwent cesarean section -A case report-
Kum Hee Chung, Jong Yeon Lee, Tong Kyun Ko, Chung Hyun Park, Duk Hee Chun, Hyeon Jeong Yang, Hyun Jue Gill, Min Ku Kim
Korean J Anesthesiol. 2010 December; 59(Suppl): S86–S89. Published online 2010 December 31. doi: 10.4097/kjae.2010.59.S.S86
PMCID:
PMC3030065
ArticlePubReaderPDF–387K

Select item 34241777.
Neurolysis for Megalgia Paresthetica
Byung-Chul Son, Deok-Ryeong Kim, Il-Sup Kim, Jae-Taek Hong, Jae-Hoon Sung, Sang-Won Lee

J Korean Neurosurg Soc. 2012 June; 51(6): 363–366. Published online 2012 June 30. doi: 10.3340/jkns.2012.51.6.363
PMCID:
PMC3424177
ArticlePubReaderPDF–539K

Select item 26151458.
Prone Position-Related **Meralgia** Paresthetica after Lumbar Spinal Surgery : A Case Report and Review of the Literature
Keun-Tae Cho, Ho Jun Lee
J Korean Neurosurg Soc. 2008 December; 44(6): 392–395. Published online 2008 December 31. doi: 10.3340/jkns.2008.44.6.392
PMCID:
PMC2615145
ArticlePubReaderPDF–236K

Select item 26149579.
Persistent bilateral anterior hip pain in a young adult due to **meralgia** paresthetica: a case report
Vijay D Shetty, Gautam M Shetty
Cases J. 2008; 1: 396. Published online 2008 December 15. doi: 10.1186/1757-1626-1-396
PMCID:
PMC2614957
ArticlePubReaderPDF–280K

Select item 196427810.
Meralgia paraesthetica--an addition to
'seatbelt syndrome'.
Stephen M. Blake, Nicholas J. Treble
Ann R Coll Surg Engl. 2004 November;
86(6): W6–W7.
PMCID:
PMC1964278
SummaryPDF–100K

Select item 249301611.
Case Report: **Meralgia** Paresthetica in a
Baseball Pitcher
Kenichi Otoshi, Yoshiyasu Itoh, Akihito
Tsujino, Shinichi Kikuchi
Clin Orthop Relat Res. 2008 September;
466(9): 2268–2270. Published online 2008
May 29. doi: 10.1007/s11999-008-0307-3
PMCID:
PMC2493016
ArticlePubReaderPDF–181K

Select item 138565912.
AN OSTEOPLASTIC NEUROLYSIS
OPERATION FOR THE CURE OF
MERALGIA PARESTHETICA
Ferdinand C. Lee
Ann Surg. 1941 January; 113(1): 85–94.
PMCID:

PMC1385659
Summarypage Browsepdf–912K

Select item 335868613.
Femoral Neuropathy and **Meralgia**
Paresthetica Secondary to an Iliacus
Hematoma
Tae Im Yi, Tae Hee Yoon, Joo Sup Kim, Ga
Eun Lee, Bo Ra Kim
Ann Rehabil Med. 2012 April; 36(2): 273–
277. Published online 2012 April 30. doi:
10.5535/arm.2012.36.2.273
PMCID:
PMC3358686
ArticlePubReaderPDF–264K

Select item 264706414.
A manual therapy and exercise approach to
meralgia paresthetica in pregnancy: a case
report
Clayton D. Skaggs, Brett A. Winchester,
Michael Vianin, Heidi Prather
J Chiropr Med. 2006 Fall; 5(3): 92–96.
Published online 2006. doi: 10.1016/S0899-
3467(07)60140-2
PMCID:
PMC2647064
ArticlePubReaderPDF–94K

Select item 142114115.

Meralgia Paresthetica, The Elusive
Diagnosis: Clinical Experience With 14 Adult
Patients
Gregory K. Ivins
Ann Surg. 2000 August; 232(2): 281–286.
PMCID:
PMC1421141
ArticlePubReaderPDF–405K

Select item 194779916.
Meralgia paresthetica as a cause of leg
discomfort
R. K. Jones
Can Med Assoc J. 1974 September 21; 111(6):
541–542.
PMCID:
PMC1947799
SummaryPage BrowsePDF–468K

Select item 235495817.
MERALGIA PARAESTHETICA
J. Reid
Br Med J. 1916 November 4; 2(2914): 636.
PMCID:
PMC2354958
SummaryPage BrowsePDF–294K

Select item 134284918.
Abdominal aortic aneurysm presenting as
meralgia paraesthetica.

A Brett, T Hodgetts
J Accid Emerg Med. 1997 January; 14(1):
49–51.
PMCID:
PMC1342849
SummaryPage BrowsePDF–747K

Select item 185953919.
Meralgia paraesthetica--a sports lesion in
girl gymnasts.
J. Macgregor, J. A. Moncur
Br J Sports Med. 1977 April; 11(1): 16–19.
PMCID:
PMC1859539
SummaryPage BrowsePDF–987K

Made in the USA
Monee, IL
17 July 2023